Thyroid Disease: An Introduction

Dealing With Thyroid Symptoms with Diet and Treatment

By: Ashley Wells

PUBLISHERS NOTES

Disclaimer

This publication is intended to provide helpful and informative material. It is not intended to diagnose, treat, cure, or prevent any health problem or condition, nor is it intended to replace the advice of a physician. No action should be taken solely on the contents of this book. Always consult your physician or qualified health-care professional on any matters regarding your health and before adopting any suggestions in this book or drawing inferences from it.

The author and publisher specifically disclaim all responsibility for any liability, loss or risk, personal or otherwise, which is incurred as a consequence, directly or indirectly, from the use or application of any contents of this book.

Any and all product names referenced within this book are the trademarks of their respective owners. None of these owners have sponsored, authorized, endorsed, or approved this book.

Always read all information provided by the manufacturers' product labels before using their products. The author and publisher are not responsible for claims made by manufacturers.

Paperback Edition

Manufactured in the United States of America

Dedication

This book is dedicated to my mother Louisa. Through her struggle with thyroid disease, I saw how strong she truly is and I learned how to be strong as well to support her.

TABLE OF CONTENTS

Publishers Notes 2

Dedication 3

Chapter 1- The Thyroid-How Does It Work? 5

Chapter 2- Thyroid Disease-Who Does It Affect? 9

Chapter 3- Thyroid Disease-Signs and Symptoms 13

Chapter 4- Thyroid Disease-How Is It Diagnosed? 17

Chapter 5- Thyroid Disease-Treatment Options 20

Chapter 6- Thyroid Disease-Alternate Treatment Options 24

Chapter 7- Thyroid Disease-Dietary Changes To Make If You Have Been Diagnosed 28

About The Author 32

Chapter 1 - The Thyroid - How Does It Work?

The thyroid is an important endocrine gland that is responsible for many important functions within the body. The thyroid regulates the way we feel and respond to stimuli on a daily basis. If the function of the thyroid is interrupted, it can cause severe damage to the body and wreak havoc in a variety of different ways. This chapter will outline the basic information about the thyroid and its function in the body.

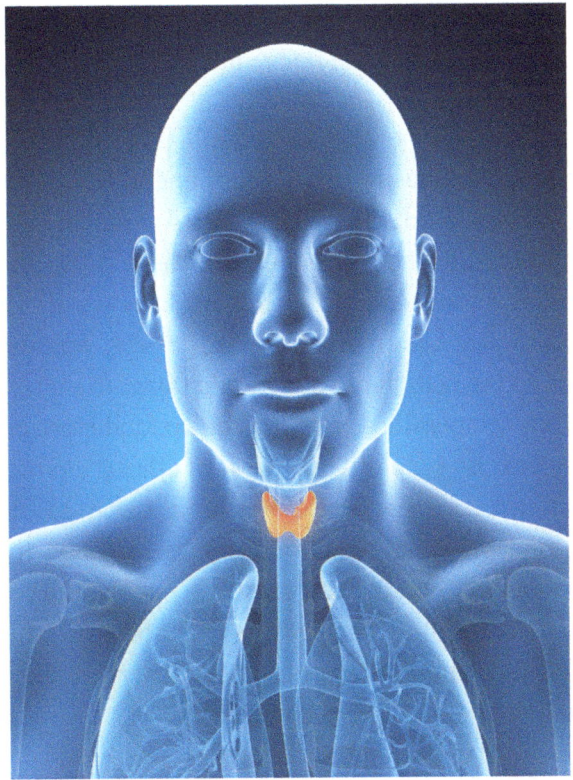

The thyroid is the largest endocrine gland in the body. It is located in the neck within the bulge that is displayed in the throats of many, commonly referred to as the Adam's apple. The thyroid is made up of two different parts that make it somewhat resemble the shape of a butterfly. The gland is covered in a thin layer that functions as a type of skin to protect it. The thyroid gland has the unique ability to change its size and shape when necessary. The gland is said to weigh, on average, 20-60 grams in healthy adults, though it typically increases in size in pregnant women.

The thyroid is the main center in the body for the direction of hormones, or tiny signals that give cells information about how to act and respond. It does this by producing two extremely important hormones called Triiodothyronine and Thyroxine (more commonly referred to as T3 and T4). The thyroid releases these important little hormones throughout the body. These hormones then give information to the cells in the body, and ultimately determine how the cells will act.

Though, overall, it helps maintain order and ensure proper bodily functions across the board, certain aspects of health can be more directly attributed to the thyroid. One of these is the metabolism. The hormones produced by the thyroid increase the metabolic rate. To increase the metabolic rate, these hormones send information to the cells in the body to do things like increase heart rate and body temperature and break down food more quickly. So, if the thyroid is sending out less of these hormones, the metabolism will slow as these functions begin to slow. And, reflexively, if more of these hormones are sent out, the rate of these functions will increase and cause the metabolism to increase. Ultimately, though the technical explanation is much more complicated it is these hormones that determine the speed at which all of the body's cells will operate.

For infants and young children, the thyroid hormones are vital for the overall development of the children, particularly brain development. The thyroid hormones also regulate the rate of physical growth and development of young people.

Additionally, these hormones will determine how the body will receive and be affected by other hormones that the body produces. T3 and T4 are like the master hormones that set the stage in the cells for the use and effectiveness of other hormones that the body will produce and disperse to those same cells. T3 and T4 will lay down the groundwork for the other hormones to be effective or ineffective within cells.

There are two main thyroid dysfunctions that can occur. These are hyperthyroidism and hypothyroidism. Hyperthyroidism is the term for a thyroid gland that is overproducing the hormones that it regulates, T3 and T4. Usually this disorder occurs in the context of the autoimmune disease, Grave's Disease in which certain antibodies begin signaling the thyroid to produce extra amounts of the hormones. This can result in a variety of complications such as thyroid growth, a rapid heart rate, eyes that protrude, muscular weakness, lethargy, diarrhea, and other symptoms.

Hypothyroidism, on the other hand, is a condition that occurs when the thyroid produces too little of the hormones T3 and T4. This could also be caused by autoimmune diseases, but additionally, could be the result of iodine deficiencies, birth defects, or a complication following an operation on the thyroid. Sufferers will typically experience weight gain and baldness and the inability to handle cold temperatures.

Other disorders include thyroid cancer and cysts that grow on the thyroid. Additionally, there is a condition called thyroiditis, in which the body begins to fight the actions of its own thyroid. This condition, however, typically begins with hyperthyroidism before other complications redefine the disorder.

Both hyperthyroidism and hypothyroidism can be treated with modern medications. However, these medications have not been

Thyroid Disease

perfected. While symptoms may be treatable, the medication procedure requires a great deal of medical monitoring and the medication may begin to lose its effect over time. Another option for those who experience hyperthyroidism is called iodine radiation. In this procedure, portions of the thyroid are carefully killed off in an attempt to decrease the amounts of the hormones that are produced. A part of the thyroid can also be removed via surgery.

Overall, the thyroid is one of the most important centers in the body. It is responsible for the production and distribution of the hormones T3 and T4. These hormones are responsible for a great deal including the general function of cells in the body. The hormones regulate the rate at which cells will function in the body. The rate at which cells function can have far reaching consequences including the rate of overall bodily development and the body's responsiveness to other hormones. There are a variety of complications that can arise in regard to the function of the thyroid. Though these can be treated to some degree, they are difficult problems to work through and can be quite serious.

Chapter 2- Thyroid Disease-Who Does It Affect?

Thyroid disease is a term that can describe several conditions that affect the thyroid. Most often it refers to hyperthyroidism or hypothyroidism, but goiters as well as thyroiditis may also be considered types of thyroid disease. As mentioned in chapter 1, the thyroid is a gland shaped somewhat like a butterfly that is responsible for making certain hormones in the body. These hormones, in turn, affect how a number of processes in the body are completed such as heart rate and even how fast calories are burned. When the thyroid does not function normally and a person suffers from a thyroid disease they exhibit a number of symptoms and there are also a number of ways to solve the issues and treat the disease. Many diseases of the thyroid are interconnected. Therefore, some thyroid diseases also lead to other thyroid diseases.

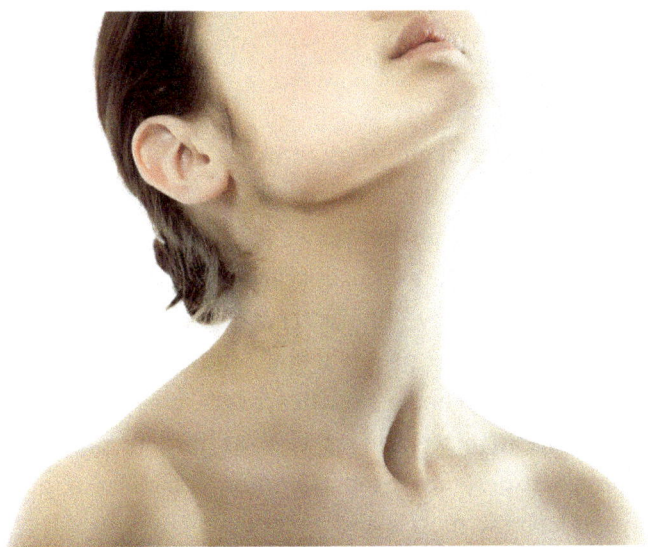

Thyroid Disease
<u>What is Hyperthyroidism?</u>

Hyperthyroidism is when the thyroid gland produces more hormones than it is supposed to. This result is a substantially increased metabolism. The symptoms can vary a great deal from person to person, but common symptoms include nervousness, mood swings, fatigue and being intolerant of heat. Some sufferers of this thyroid disease also experience hand tremors, trouble sleeping, a rapid or irregular heart rate, weight loss or diarrhea. Others may also develop a goiter, which is when the thyroid becomes enlarged and causes the neck to appear swollen.

Diagnosis requires blood tests and occasionally a thyroid scan. Treatment is typically in the form of medication. Just as the symptoms vary, no single treatment works for all patients with this condition. Sometimes radioiodine therapy is required and sometimes even surgery to repair the thyroid in order to slow it down. Removing a part of the thyroid is sometimes necessary to decrease its hormone production in severe cases.

<u>What is Hypothyroidism?</u>

Hyperthyroidism can be thought of as an overactive thyroid, while hypothyroidism is the opposite. This thyroid disease results in the thyroid not producing enough hormones for the body. It shares some of the same symptoms as its counterpart such as fatigue as well as emotional instability. Characteristic symptoms of this condition include weight gain, being intolerant of cold temperatures, constipation and a slow heart rate. It can also result in heavy menstruation in women as well as fertility problems. Sometimes people experience other symptoms such as a puffy face, dry skin and hair and muscle and joint pain.

Hypothyroidism is diagnosed with blood tests just like hyperthyroidism. Treatment involves taking a synthetic thyroid hormone in order to replace the hormones that the body is not producing on its own. The synthetic thyroid hormone is known as levothyroxine and is taken orally. It takes one to two weeks for hormone levels to stabilize in the body and for the drug's effects to be noticeable.

What is a Goiter?

Developing a goiter is the result of not having enough iodine in the diet. They are fairly uncommon in the western world due to the use of iodized salt. A lack of iodine will result in an overproduction of thyroid hormones, which causes the gland to become enlarged. It may also cause the gland to develop nodules. It is closely associated with hyperthyroidism. The swelling is not painful, but often results in a cough as well as obvious swelling in the throat and neck.

Small goiters are often left untreated if they are not causing problems and are not getting larger. Larger goiters are treated with medications similar to those used for hyperthyroidism and hypothyroidism. Treatment depends largely upon the cause of the goiter. Sometimes surgeries are necessary and involve removing all or part of the thyroid gland. If the thyroid gland is removed hormone therapy is required for the rest of the patients' life because they often develop hypothyroidism.

What is Thyroiditis?

Thyroiditis can be caused by a number of factors. There are also several forms of thyroiditis including Hashimoto's Disease, which is an autoimmune condition, and Riedel's thyroiditis, which is another disease that is believed to be autoimmune related as well. The disease can also be the result of taking certain medications and postpartum thyroiditis occurs in some women after giving birth. Treatment depends upon the cause of the condition. Riedel's thyroiditis is a chronic condition with no cure. Having any form of thyroiditis puts one at risk for both hyperthyroidism as well as hypothyroidism.

Who Does Thyroid Disease Affect?

Hyperthyroidism and hypothyroidism are both more common in women than men and more common in people over sixty years of age, but anyone at any time can technically develop either condition because there are so many possible causes. There are a number of risk factors that will increase your chances too. Grave's Disease or other autoimmune conditions are the most common cause of hyperthyroidism. Grave's Disease often runs in families as does hyperthyroidism. It may also be the result of consuming high amounts of iodine or having thyroiditis. Thyroiditis most often results in hypothyroidism.

Hypothyroidism can be caused by another autoimmune disorder, Hashimoto's Disease, but it can also be congenital and tends to run in families as well. It may also be the result of thyroid surgeries in which part of the thyroid is removed, such as with thyroid cancer or even hyperthyroidism. Some medications may also cause the thyroid to produce too few hormones. Pregnant women or women that were pregnant within the last six months are also at higher risk of developing hypothyroidism due to their higher risk of developing postpartum thyroiditis.

Chapter 3- Thyroid Disease-Signs and Symptoms

As I noted, the thyroid is a gland located in the neck and it is shaped like a butterfly. The main purpose of the thyroid is to control the body's metabolism. Around 59 million people suffer from thyroid problems; however, most people who suffer from thyroid problems do not know it. When a person has a thyroid problem and it goes undiagnosed, it can lead to obesity, heart disease, anxiety, hair loss, depression, sexual dysfunction, and infertility. The reason thyroid disease often goes undiagnosed is because people do not know the signs and symptoms of thyroid disease. Many people will experience symptoms and chalk them up to something else.

As I mentioned in Chapter 2, in most cases of thyroid problems, a person will have an overactive thyroid (hyperthyroidism) or an under active thyroid (hypothyroidism). When the thyroid is overactive, the body's metabolism is working too fast and when the thyroid is under active, the body's metabolism slows down to a dangerous rate.

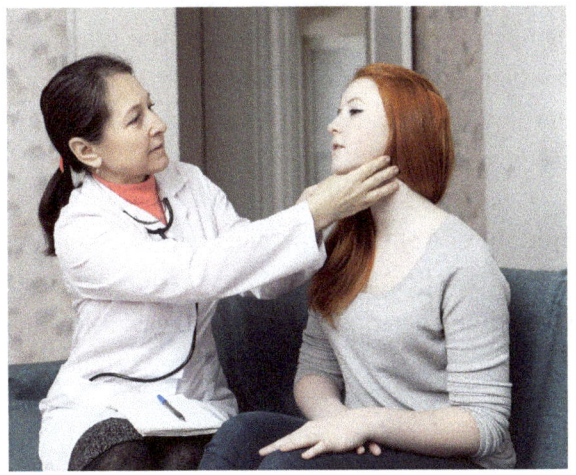

Thyroid Disease
Some people with thyroid disease will experience muscle and joint pain. Moving the elbows and the knees can become very painful. They may also develop carpel tunnel syndrome in the hands, tarsal tunnel in the legs, and plantars fasclitis in the feet. When a person develops these symptoms, the last thing that they think of is thyroid disease.

When a person develops a goiter, an enlarged thyroid gland, it is a sign that he/she may have thyroid disease. The symptoms of goiter are swelling of the neck, discomfort when wearing turtlenecks or neckties, or a hoarse voice. One very obvious symptom of goiter is a visibly enlarged thyroid gland. These are all symptoms of thyroid disease.

When a person has a thyroid problem, he/she can experience problems with his/her hair and skin. When a person suffers from hypothyroidism, his/her hair can become dry, brittle, coarse, and break easily and fall out. He/she may also notice hair loss on the outer edges of the eyebrows. The skin of a person with hypothyroidism can become very thick, dry, and scaly. When a person has hyperthyroidism, his/her hair loss can be very severe. His/her skin will become very fragile and thin. When a person with thyroid disease experiences these symptoms, he/she will think that it is the shampoo that he/she are using, or the soap, and even the styling tools that he/she use on his/her hair. A thyroid problem is typically the last thing that he/she suspects is causing these hair and skin issues.

When people suffer from hypothyroidism, they can have problems with long term constipation. This constipation can even be very severe. When other persons have hyperthyroidism, they can get diarrhea quite often, and in many cases, they can develop irritable bowel syndrome (IBS).

Women can show signs of thyroid disease during their menstrual periods. When a woman suffers from hypothyroidism, she will have a much heavier and more painful period than she is used to. When a woman has hyperthyroidism, she will experience lighter and less frequent periods. In some cases, women with an overactive thyroid will not have a period at all. In cases of long term, undiagnosed thyroid disease, it can cause infertility which can be devastating for women who want to have children.

When a person's cholesterol level is not normal, it can be a sign of thyroid disease. When a person has high cholesterol, the doctor will recommend a change in diet and also recommend a daily exercise regimen. In some cases, a cholesterol lowering medication will also be prescribed. If a person is doing everything that the doctor recommended and there is still no change in cholesterol, chances are the thyroid can be causing the cholesterol problem. Hypothyroidism can cause cholesterol problems which cannot be rectified by diet, exercise, or medication. When a person is suffering from hyperthyroidism, they may have low cholesterol. Like the other symptoms of thyroid disease, these symptoms may be thought to be the result of another condition.

When a person becomes suddenly depressed for no reason, it can be a symptom of hypothyroidism. Many doctors will not look to hypothyroidism at first. They will prescribe an anti-depressant and hope that the patient begins to feel better. When a person is depressed and has hypothyroidism, the anti-depressants will not always work. When a person suffers from hyperthyroidism, they can develop anxiety and the sudden onset of a panic disorder. Like depression, most doctors will not immediately turn to thyroid disease due to depression and anxiety. It could take one or more of the other symptoms to put it all together.

Thyroid Disease
Weight problems are one of the most common and recognized symptoms. When a person is eating a low calorie diet and exercising daily and still fails to lose weight, chances are he/she is suffering from hypothyroidism. Because his/her thyroid is working too slowly, his/her metabolism is working slow making it difficult for it to burn calories. When a person has not changed his/her diet or exercise regimen in anyway and are still losing a good deal of weight, hyperthyroidism could be the reason. When the thyroid is working overtime, so is the body's metabolism burning calories at a very high rate. When a patient goes to the doctor with weight issues, thyroid disease usually comes to mind first.

Feeling fatigued is a sign of a thyroid problem. If a person is getting a full 8 to 10 hours of sleep at night and he/she is still tired all day and cannot get through the day without a nap, hypothyroidism could be the reason why. When a person suffers from hyperthyroidism, they may not be able to sleep at night, leaving them tired during the day.

If you have one or more of these symptoms, it is important that you go see the doctor so that blood tests can be done to test the activity of your thyroid. Allowing thyroid disease to go untreated can lead to long term problems.

Chapter 4- Thyroid Disease-How Is It Diagnosed?

Just like any disease, the diagnosis of Thyroid disease follows several stages. The first and most important is to see if the symptoms one is experiencing are typical for thyroid disease patients. The next step is to look at associated factors; these may include environmental, nutritional, lifestyle and family medical history. Once such factors are reviewed, doctors will decide on tests like blood, imaging, tissue/cell testing (biopsy) or a simple clinical observation/evaluation. Additional tests might be run, but most of the thyroid diseases types will easily be diagnosed under these tests. It is important to mention that today, patients have the option of conducting self-tests, before running and seeking qualifying evaluations from their medical providers. This chapter seeks to review the different tests, or diagnosis methods for common thyroid diseases, problems.

During clinical evaluation, your doctor will ask typical questions most doctors ask during a medical visit. They do so to try and confirm or corroborate their evaluation. They will also ask such questions to understand what they can't observe, feel or test. When evaluating for Thyroid disease, they will palpate or touch gently under your neck to feel the thyroid. They will most likely place their stethoscope on your thyroid and listen. Since Thyroid disease affects the normal functioning of the nervous system, they will conduct a knee-jerk test also called reflex test. They will also look at other major areas, including your heart, blood-pressure, your nails and especially the largest external organ; your skin. Because Thyroid disease may include a puffy face, thinning hair, dry skin and painful or swollen joints. The doctor will pay quite some attention to these areas. Other questions the doctor may ask include your bowel movement texture, your sensitivity to weather elements and off course, your energy levels. They will also look at the history of your weight and for women; they will also inquire about your menstrual flow history.

Once a doctor is convinced that there is need for further tests, they could order for a simple blood test or advanced tests depending on the symptoms they are looking to separate. These tests will mostly be checking for two hormones; Thyroxine commonly called T4 and Triiodothyronine simply called T3. These two hormones are produced by the Thyroid gland and are crucial for the basic organ functions in muscles, growth, circulation and nerves. The blood tests will check for total T4's and T3's. It will also check for free T4's and free T3's. They may also test for antibodies for the following; thyroid peroxidase, Antithyroid Microsomal, Thyroglobulin, and Thyroid Receptor Antibodies. They also check for Resin Uptake also called TR3U and for TBG's or Thyroid Binding Globulin. Your doctor will test for any of these to check for anomalies in the expected levels. This will help them disqualify or qualify any clinical evaluation they already have. They will also be able to separate the nature of the thyroid disease if you have one. Depending on the quantities, presence or absence of any of the elements above, the doctor will observe if it's Hypothyroidism or otherwise.

The doctor might want to further see if there are additional causes for your thyroid disease, or thyroid disease symptoms. They have the choice of running different types of imaging. A simple CT scan and or nuclear scan may be employed to help identify obvious Thyroid issues like goiter, enlarged thyroid nodules Thyroiditis. A thyroid ultrasound can be run to check for tissue or fluid-filled cysts. A regular Magnetic resonance imaging, commonly called RMI can also be used to check for any discrepancies on the shape of Thyroid gland. Additional tests can be performed again, all these are meant to reinforce or separate observations obtained from both blood and clinical tests.

The doctor might need to use FNA or Fine Needle Aspirations to collect cells or tissue for cancer testing. Depending on the discoveries through imaging, the doctor will decide on the suitable point to collect the tissue, and seventy-five percent of the time, this test will be able to give a correct result. The doctor will inspect the cells or tissue for cancer or the autoimmune disease; Hashimoto's thyroiditis. A few other tests that are acceptable but not very popular include saliva and urinary testing. An iodine path test or even testing basal body temperature can help point patients towards identifying if further thyroid tests might be necessary.

Finally, the personal test-yourself kits available are based on checking for T3's, T4's and the reverse for the same. These test-kits could also be used to check for microsomal and thyroid peroxidase antibodies. It is key to mention that for all tests, the most important aspect is physical evaluation and for this a "Thyroid check-neck" is right at your disposal. Here is a simple procedure that you can perform by following simple steps: Get a glass of water, stand before a mirror and stretch your neck towards the back, take a gulp of water and swallow keenly observing the area above the collar bone and below the Adam's Apple. If you notice any enlargement or swelling in that area, repeat all the steps and confirm the bump or swelling by touch. If you confirm your previous observation, call your doctor and get checked. Remember, in medicine, you are better-off being over-cautious.

Chapter 5 - Thyroid Disease - Treatment Options

Millions of people in the U.S. remain undiagnosed for thyroid disease every year. This disease is a treatable and highly curable disease. Most cases are controlled with daily medication or a combination of medications. In extreme cases, surgery may be required. The treatment of thyroid disease is directly dependent on the type of thyroid disease that the patient has been afflicted with and the progression of the disease.

The thyroid releases hormones meant to deliver energy to the body's cells from the thyroid gland. This gland is located at the lower part of the neck, and it resembles a butterfly. This gland controls many functions throughout the body including sexual function, heartbeat, and moods. When not producing enough or when producing too much hormone, it causes problems with the patient's health. Warning signs of thyroid disease include moodiness, lack of energy, or mental fogginess. The thyroid gland affects different areas and functions of the body, therefore the treatment will be dependent on the type of thyroid malfunction that is occurring.

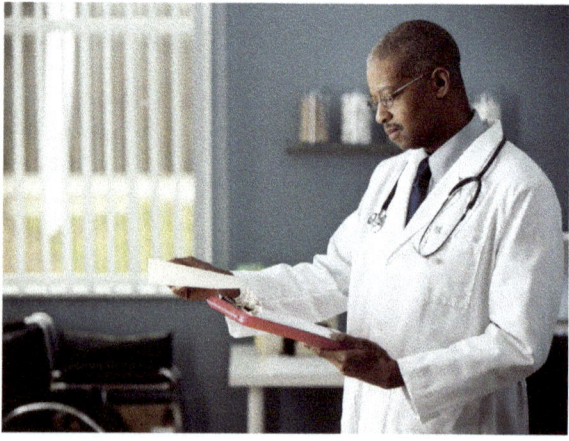

Ashley Wells
Hypothyroidism

As mentioned in Chapter 3, this condition of the thyroid gland is when it is underactive and not producing enough hormones. The cause of this condition is usually Hashimoto's disease. It attacks the autoimmune system by shutting down the thyroid gland's ability to produce the proper level of hormones. Symptoms of hypothyroidism include depression, weight gain, fatigue, and a slowing of the metabolism. The most commonly prescribed drug for the treatment of this disease is levothyroxine.

Hyperthyroidism

Grave's disease is the most common cause of the autoimmune condition called hyperthyroidism. The antibodies target the thyroid and cause it to increase hormone production. These antibodies either attack and destroy the thyroid or cause it to become overactive. The medications used to treat and manage this type of thyroid disease are drug therapy, RAI or radioactive iodine treatment, or in severe cases, surgery is necessary. Testing is done to determine which type of hyperthyroidism is present and medical treatment targeted to the specific disease.

Goiter

Goiters and nodules are lumps that form in the thyroid area in the neck. These nodules are common. Many doctors will choose to monitor the nodules and prescribe hormone replacement drugs to stop, shrink, or slow the progression of the growth. When these nodules or goiters become a cosmetic or physical problem, the physician may choose to treat the abnormalities with radioactive iodine or surgery in severe cases.

Thyroid Disease
<u>Thyroid Cancer</u>

This cancer is rather uncommon among the list of human cancers. The survival rates for this type of cancer are high, with results of 95% of all patients having a long survival rate with no reoccurrence. This disease of the malignant thyroid nodules or tissue has four distinct types of cancer associated with it.

Papillary Cancer is the most common among the thyroid cancers. The thyroid contains numerous papillaries therefore making them a larger target for disease. This type of cancer usually involves only one side of the gland, and sometimes will spread to the lymph nodes. Although this cancer is the most common, it is highly curable.

Follicular Cancer is involving the follicles of the thyroid. These follicles are responsible for the growth and development of tissues. If this type of cancer spreads, it usually infects the arteries and veins of the gland and more distant areas such as the bone, skin, lung, etc. The long-term survival rates are good for this type of cancer although it is more common in older patients.

Medullary Thyroid Cancer is usually found in the center of the upper lobe of the thyroid. This type of cancer spreads to the lymph nodes. This type of cancer comes from the cells that produce the hormone calcitonin rather than the cells that produce the thyroid hormones. Genetics play a part in the occurrence of this type of cancer, which is also highly curable.

Anaplastic Cancer is the most invasive and progressive form of thyroid cancer. This type of cancer can spread to the lymph nodes as well as to other organs. Most cases are discovered by a lump or bulging of the neck. This type of cancer is mostly found in men over the age of 65, and the success rate for cure is much lower than that of the other forms of thyroid cancer.

Thyroid cancer is often treated with different medications or surgery. There are medications such as levothyroxine that target the nodules to eliminate them slowly over time. In some cases, it may be necessary to treat the patient with radioactive iodine. In most cases when cancer is involved in the thyroid, the thyroid is surgically removed.

Thyroiditis

This type of disease involves the inflammation of the thyroid gland. There are different specific types of thyroiditis such as painless or silent, Riedel's, Postpartum, or acute infectious thyroiditis. These conditions involve a physician taking samples, draining fluids, and antibiotic therapy depending on the results from the fluid samples. In rare cases, the doctor may call for the mass to be surgically removed.

The treatment of most thyroid diseases involves the administering of antibiotic medications. These medications either alone or in combination with other medications are meant to shrink the infected mass or eliminate it completely. Most people respond well to medication, but in extreme cases, some patients have to undergo surgery. Thyroid disease is a highly undiagnosed disease among Americans, but it is also a very highly curable disease. As with all forms of cancer, early detection is the key to longevity.

Chapter 6- Thyroid Disease- Alternate Treatment Options

As mentioned throughout the book, the thyroid is a gland in the neck whose job it is to help regulate a wide variety of body functions, from metabolism to breathing to hormone production. When someone has a thyroid disease, whether it's cancer or simply an imbalance, it's important to get that treated quickly. For those who want to try to avoid traditional medicines though, or who would like to at least attempt a more holistic approach, there are a variety of different things that can be done to treat thyroid disease depending on the individual, his or her health, and the nature of the thyroid disease in question.

You Are What You Eat

One of the most common alternative forms of treatment for a thyroid condition is to alter someone's diet. And, while there have been a lot of different articles claiming there is one food or another that represents a miracle cure for everything from cancer to hypothyroidism, it's important to take all of that hype with a few grains of salt.

There are some foods that those with thyroid conditions should avoid. Soy is top of that list, as it's been shown to have at least a mild negative effect on a person's thyroid gland. There have also been claims that coconut oil is a necessity for helping regulate the thyroid; these are half-truths at best. In some instances adding coconut oil to one's diet can have beneficial effects, but that will not always be the case.

In order to determine what someone needs to do to improve his or her diet to control a thyroid condition it's important to speak to a professional. A doctor who specializes in thyroid treatments and the effect that diet can have on a condition will be able to give an individual a detailed plan for altering his or her diet in such a way that it will help control the thyroid condition. This could involve simple instructions such as cutting out caffeine, alcohol, and processed foods, or it could be a more elaborate diet plan based on that individual's particular needs. Generally speaking though, an individual who suffers from a thyroid condition is going to want a diet that is low in carbohydrates, which has a high amount of protein, and which contains all of the healthy, fatty acids that a person can get his or her hands on in order to keep that person's body chemistry and thyroid gland balanced.

Exercise

While it might seem a little overly simplistic, exercise is one of the biggest forms of alternative treatment for thyroid conditions. Because a regular workout regimen helps regulate the body, it can often help even out problems with one's thyroid. It can also help regulate weight, which is a major problem that those with thyroid disease often have.

The kinds of exercise which are best will depend on an individual's needs, and the sort of physical fitness he or she already possesses. One of the most commonly recommended exercise treatments for those who have a thyroid condition however is yoga. Yoga can be learned and mastered by anyone no matter what the person's level of fitness is, and the balance of both mental and physical can often help alleviate problems caused by thyroid disease. While yoga is not a cure, nor is most exercise, following a regular routine does help an individual with a thyroid problem keep his or her body more regulated. Keeping the condition under control is often the best someone can ask for when it comes to alternative forms of treatment.

Thyroid Disease
Herbal Supplements

While they aren't for everyone, some individuals with thyroid diseases use herbal supplements to try to help control their conditions. Primrose oil, bladderwrack and bugleweed are some of the most common herbs found in supplements for thyroid problems. Seaweed kelp and spirulina are also recommended for those dealing with thyroid disease because they are high in iodine, which is necessary for helping to produce and regulate the excretions that come from the thyroid gland. Again, it's important that anyone who plans to use an herbal supplement contact his or her doctor and get an expert opinion before trying to control a condition by his or herself. Sometimes herbs might work, but sometimes a person's body chemistry is just not what those herbs were meant to handle.

A Combination Approach

When it comes to handling and controlling a thyroid issue, a plan is typically more than the sum of its parts. Individuals who are serious about fighting their disease and maintaining a balance with their thyroid glands will embrace not just one approach, but a variety of them as a way to cover all of the bases. For instance, someone may begin a new exercise regimen, make small, gradual changes to his or her diet, and start taking an herbal supplement just to top it all off.

By combining the methods for controlling and dealing with a thyroid disease an individual increases his or her chances of finding a method that works. Because everyone's bodies are different and as such everyone's particular thyroid diseases are unique, the treatment methods will work differently for different sufferers. It's also important to remember that alternative methods are not the only answer. Often times when an alternative method like diet or exercise is combined with a medication, the results are also more than either would have achieved individually. Finding the ideal combination of treatments is what is required in order for someone to truly combat a thyroid condition.

Chapter 7- Thyroid Disease- Dietary Changes To Make If You Have Been Diagnosed

When diagnosed with a medical condition resulting from an overactive or under active thyroid gland one of the main issues facing the majority of people is what kind of food to eat to keep their thyroid gland healthy. As you have seen throughout this book, this small gland found in the lower neck is important in controlling metabolism as well as ensuring that the food we eat is converted within the body correctly to support the general health of a person. One of the first major steps to take when diagnosed with thyroid disease is to begin to eat a balanced diet, free of processed foods that can be high in fats that are difficult for the body to work off through exercise.

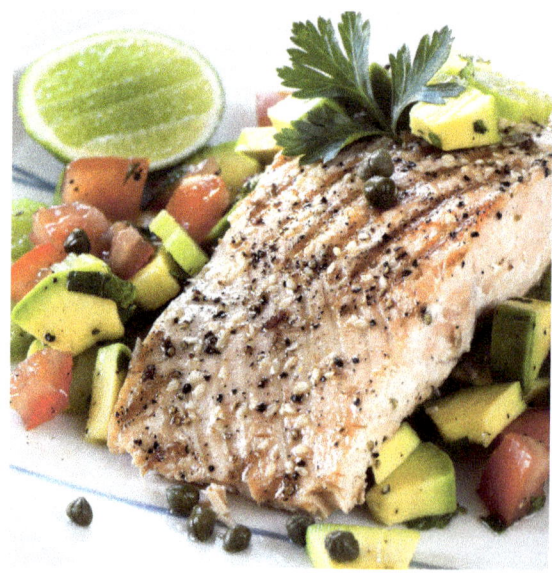

The thyroid gland is the only part of the human body capable of and required to absorb iodine. Without the correct amount of iodine, the thyroid gland will either produce too little or too much of the T3 and T4 hormones that help keep our bodies healthy. The most common way of absorbing iodine into the body is to use iodized salt when cooking and to season food. Governments around the world introduced iodizing programs for salt production to try to limit the effects of iodine deficiency. However, iodized salt is heavily processed and is therefore often ignored by many people seeking to live a healthier lifestyle. This has led to a rise in those with thyroid problems caused by a deficiency in iodine. Trace elements of iodine can be found in a variety of foods, such as seaweed, low fat milk, eggs, turkey and prunes.

Plant based foods and vegetables have now been linked to the condition known as an enlarged thyroid gland, which results in the thyroid becoming swollen as it tries to battle the chemicals found in goitrogens. This form of food can interfere with the work of the thyroid and limit the production of the T3 and T4 hormones as the gland tries to combat the harmful chemicals invading it. For those diagnosed with an enlarged thyroid the foods to be avoided include cruciferous vegetables, such as Brussels sprouts, and some root vegetables like turnips and swedes.

The all-important traces of iodine found in some fish makes it the perfect food to eat for those diagnosed with thyroid disease. Omega-3 fatty acids have long been known about as an important part of heart health and general well-being for each and every person in the world looking to live a long, healthy life. Increasing the amount of Omega-3 fatty acids, which are found in oily fish, seeds, nuts and some oils can be a good dietary change for those with an underperforming thyroid gland. Absorbing more Omega-3 fatty acids has been shown in some studies to increase the performance of the thyroid gland and make the cells of the body more liable to absorb higher levels of T3 and T4 that help to burn calories and fats.

Thyroid Disease

The thyroid is a very sensitive gland within the body and requires all around good health to ensure it functions well and keeps our body healthy as we move through our lives. Thyroid disease, in its many forms can resemble a number of other illnesses and diseases, making it hard for medical professionals to spot. The level of trace metals found in the body can often have a great impact on the level of performance a thyroid gland works at; heavy metals, zinc and copper are vital to retaining a properly performing thyroid gland. A thyroid gland producing too little of the required hormones for good health can be assisted by eating larger amounts of the cancer fighting vegetable spinach, which is high in these trace metals. Other foods that can give the thyroid a helping hand by increasing the levels of trace metals include liver and mushrooms.

The list of foods that can interfere with the proper working of the thyroid gland is long. Thiocyanate is another chemical found in a large number of foods that can quickly and easily block the passage of iodine traveling to the thyroid gland and diminish the production of the required hormones for a healthy body to be maintained. This chemical is found in corn, bamboo, broccoli and kale, and many other healthy vegetables. Because of problem of vegetables containing chemicals that compete for absorption into the thyroid gland with iodine, the person with the medical condition must make a decision on how best to treat their thyroid condition. Healthy vegetables are a recommended part of a daily balanced diet, which is also a recommended part of any healthy thyroid based diet. Many people with a thyroid condition determine the best action is to continue eating vegetables containing Thiocyanate and supplement their diet with extra amounts of iodized salt or iodine containing foods.

A popular way of avoiding many of the problems found with vegetables containing thyroid gland affecting chemicals is to eat cruciferous vegetables raw and in small amounts. The same can be done with the long list of vegetables containing Thiocyanate, whose effect is minimized when the vegetables are not cooked. Because corn and grains have been linked to problems with the thyroid gland one of the major new dietary changes many people make is to choose a gluten free diet. Cutting out foods that contain gluten can mean removing bread from a diet or switching to a gluten free product.

About The Author

Ashley Wells watched her mom battle with thyroid disease for years. To be able to help her mother, she made the decision that she had to learn all that she could about the disease. From her research she was able to anticipate what would happen next and help her mother get through it.

She was always encouraged as a child to be strong and to find the positive side of a negative situation. This is why she was not daunted when she had to find out more about her mother's condition. She encourages her readers to do same.

www.ingramcontent.com/pod-product-compliance
Ingram Content Group UK Ltd.
Pitfield, Milton Keynes, MK11 3LW, UK
UKHW022119230426
12048UKWH00010BA/608